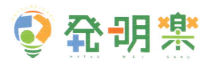

Prologue

Find your own invention!

One day, in 2007, while designing a new endoscope I realized that skill is more important than talent when it comes to inventing new things. An invention is created using several techniques in combination. I divied these techniques into four types, and named them "the four inventive skills" that can lead to the creation of a new invention : 1. Addition, 2. Subtraction, 3. Multiplication, and 4. Division. If these skills are utilized effectively, the possibilities of innovation are endless.

I wrote this book hoping that the readers will want to create inventions, or have a big dream to turn their ideas into products that would help people. The future of the whole world will be shaped by the minds of next generations. Let me show you the wonders of invention.

March 29, 2019

Masaru UEKI

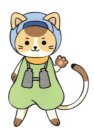

Curious Calico Cat
Innovator Mei's cat.
He is curious about everything around him and often brings Invent Rabbit his findings.

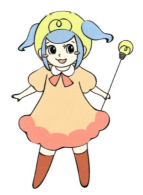

Innovator Mei
A fourth grader who wants to make people's lives easier by implementing Invent Rabbit's ideas into practice.

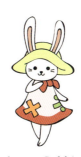

Invent Rabbit
Innovator Mei's rabbit.
She is good at creating inventions from Curious Calico Cat's findings.

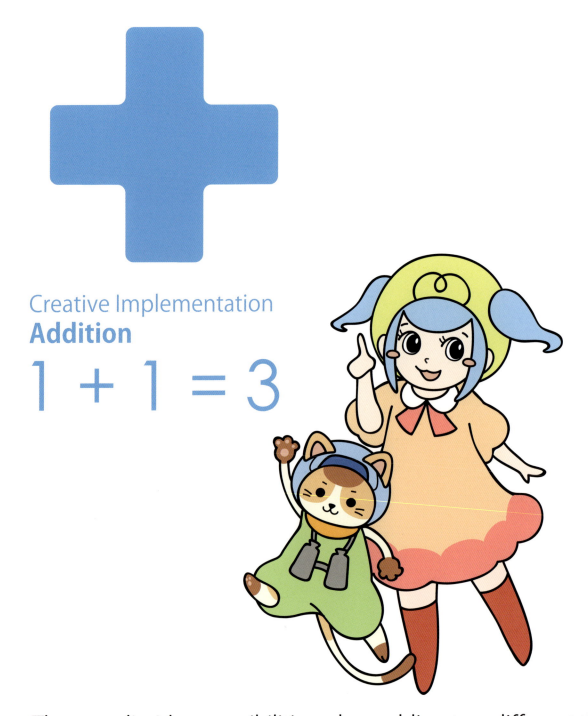

Creative Implementation
Addition
1 + 1 = 3

There are limitless possibilities when adding two different things
Combine two (or more) objects into one to add a different quality.

When something needs to be erased, an eraser is usually not at hand...

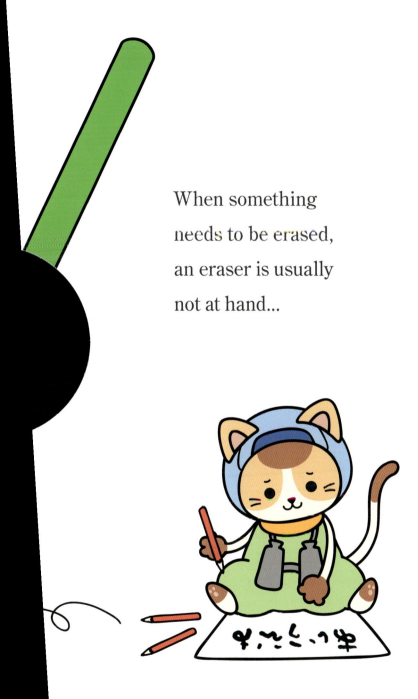

Addition – Creative Implementation "In the

✚ Invention of the **Magnifying**

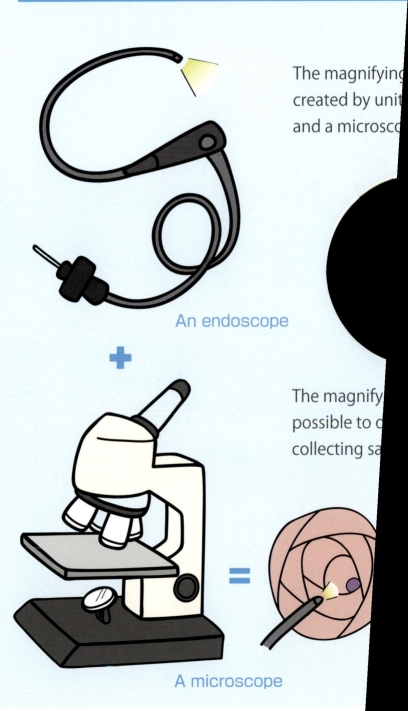

The magnifying
created by unit
and a microsco

An endoscope

The magnify
possible to c
collecting sa

A microscope

Eraser ✢ Pencil

⇒ **Pencil with attached eraser**

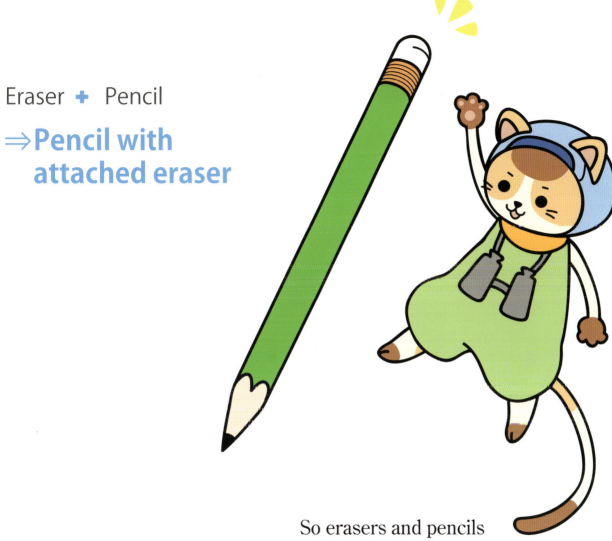

So erasers and pencils were combined! It solved the problem of searching for an eraser.

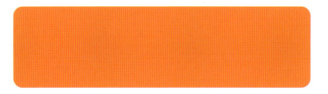

Efficient Streaming
Subtraction

1 - 0.5 = 3

Subtracting = Minimalizing

Minimalizing and taking out one of the elements from something can result in creating a totally new effect.

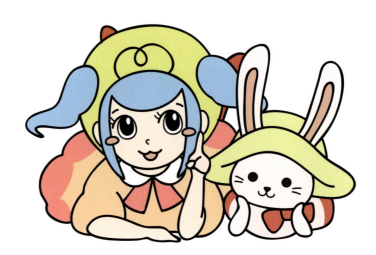

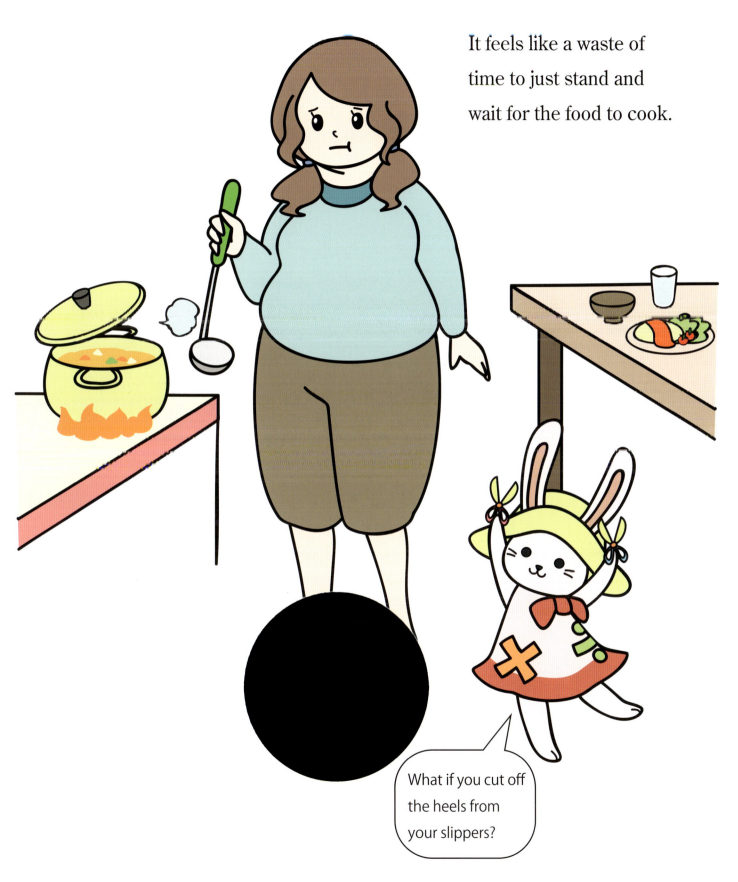

Subtraction – Efficient Streaming "In the medical field"

— Invention of the **Nasal Endoscope**

A thin endoscope slides through the nostrils without touching the throat, preventing further discomfort such as gagging.

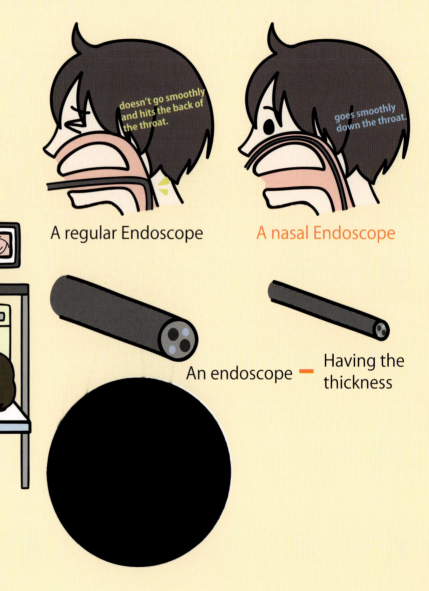

A regular Endoscope — doesn't go smoothly and hits the back of the throat.

A nasal Endoscope — goes smoothly down the throat.

An endoscope — Having the thickness

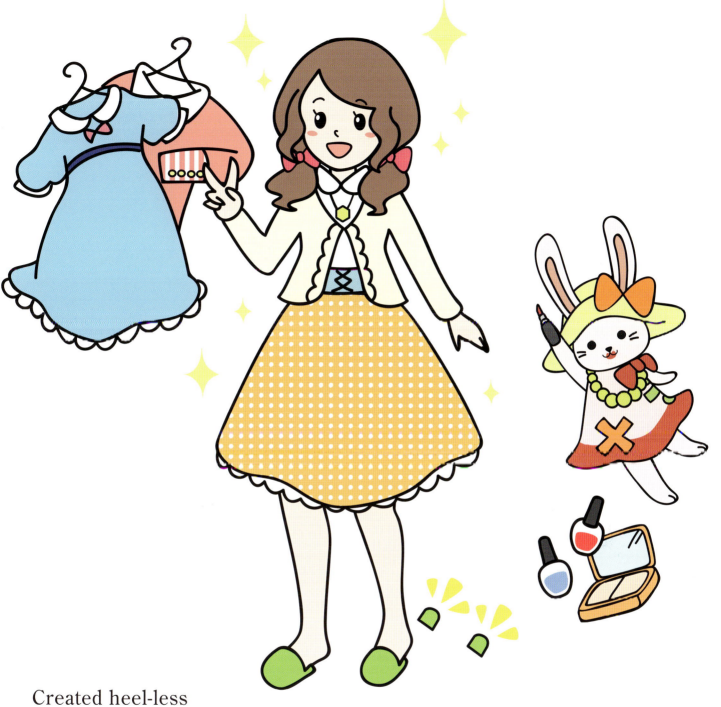

Created heel-less slippers which helped me to lose weight. Now I have more confidence to wear what I want!

Slippers — Heels
⇒ **Fitness Footwear**

Lateral Thinking **Multiplication**

1 ⇒ A

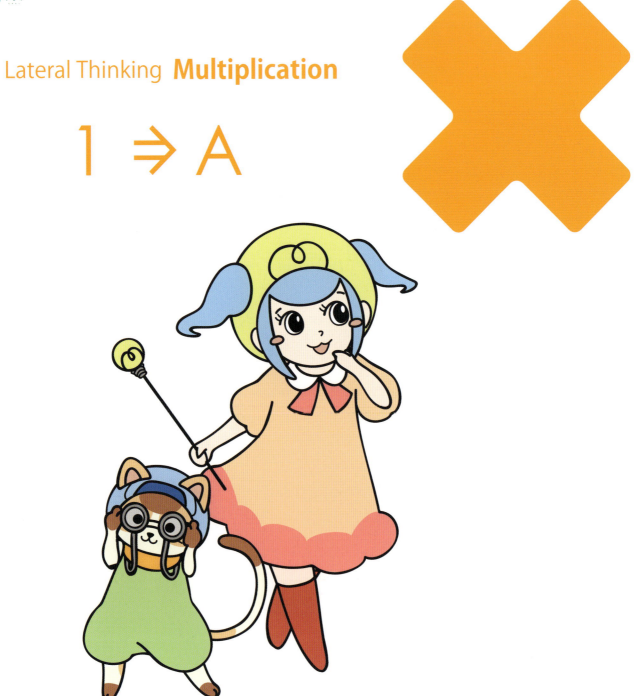

Multiplying = Recreating something in a different field

Use an idea in a new environment.

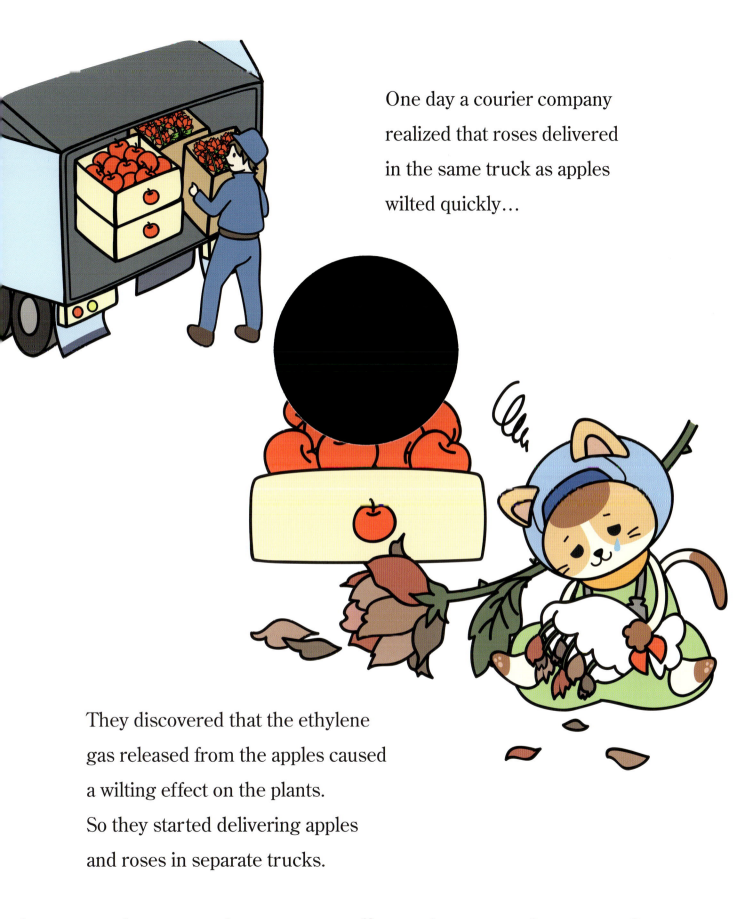

One day a courier company realized that roses delivered in the same truck as apples wilted quickly…

They discovered that the ethylene gas released from the apples caused a wilting effect on the plants. So they started delivering apples and roses in separate trucks.

Multiplication – Lateral Thinking "In the medical field"

Invention of **Ultrasonography**

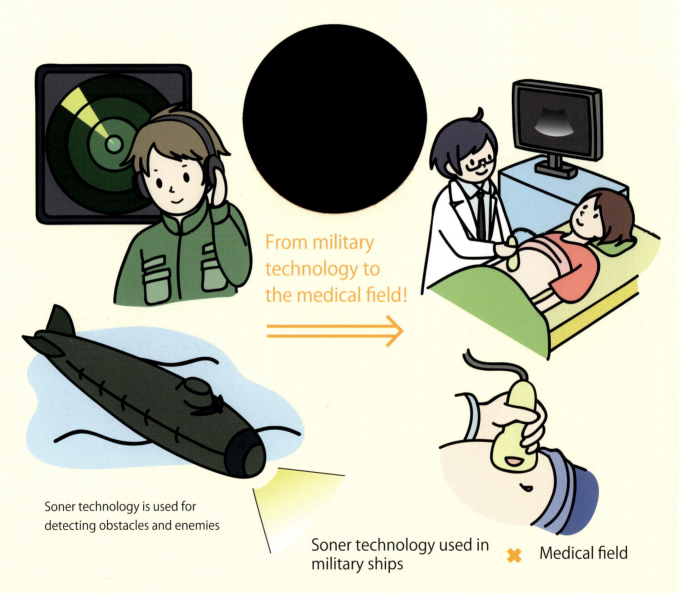

From military technology to the medical field!

Soner technology is used for detecting obstacles and enemies

Soner technology used in military ships

Medical field

Ultrasonography was developed from the sonar technology used in military ships.

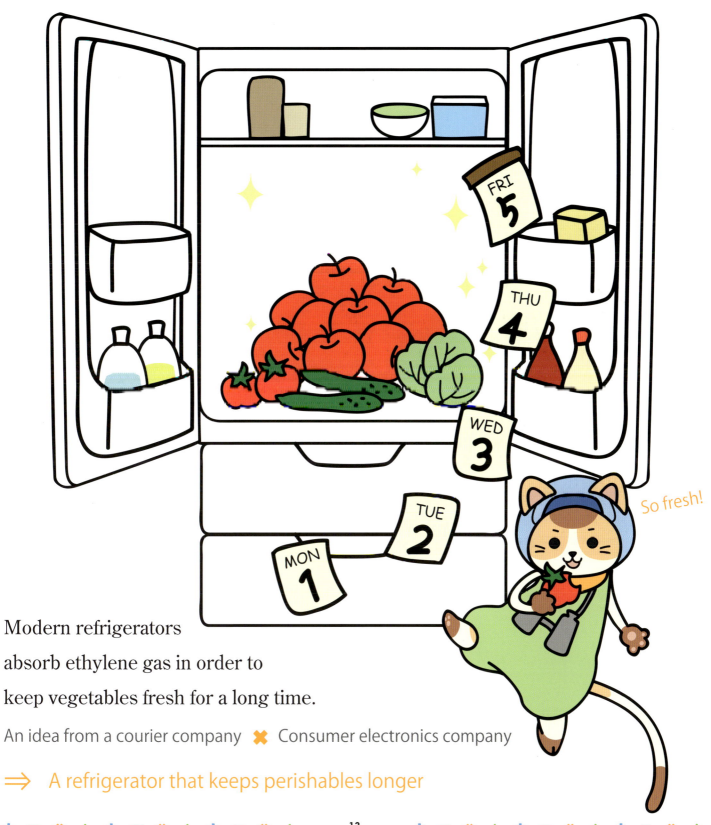

Modern refrigerators absorb ethylene gas in order to keep vegetables fresh for a long time.

An idea from a courier company ✖ Consumer electronics company

⇒ A refrigerator that keeps perishables longer

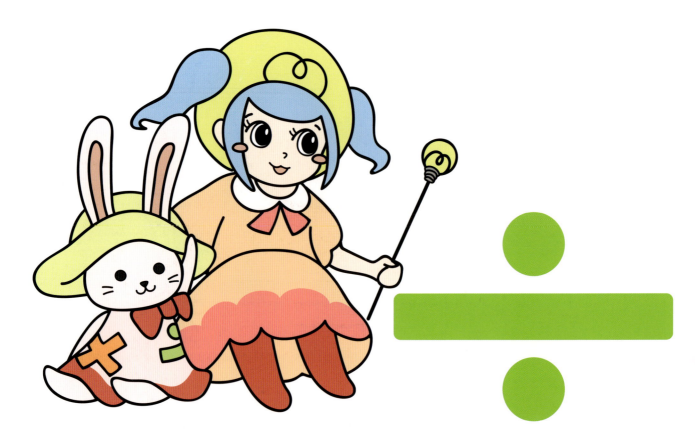

1／A

Overturns conventional wisdom
Division

Dividing = Re-evaluating

One mistake could provide more opportunities for innovation than would one successful answer.

There is value in looking at things from a different perspective. This paradigm shift in thinking could lead to new outcomes and possibilities.

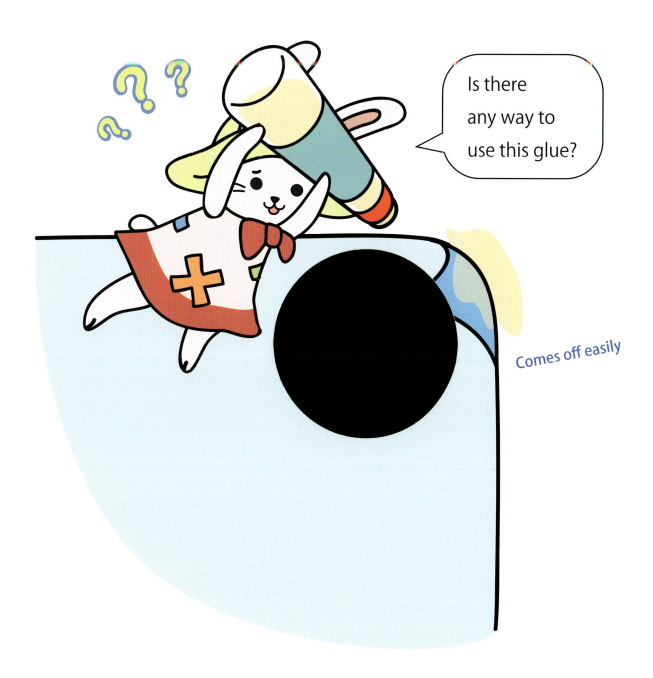

An attempt to develop a new adhesive product
that could not be detached resulted in a weaker glue.
It was a complete failure...

Division – Problem Solving "In the medical field"

÷ Invention of Artery Embolization Treatment

Arteries must not be clogged (A convention)

Treatment of cancer by clogging arteries

In 1977 Dr. Yamada (a Tottori University graduate) started a new cancer treatment. He intentionally clogged an artery to kill cancer cells. This went against conventional operations where arteries are cleared in order to circulate blood in the body. Dr. Yamada's new idea was developed into artery embolization treatment for hepatocellular carcinoma.

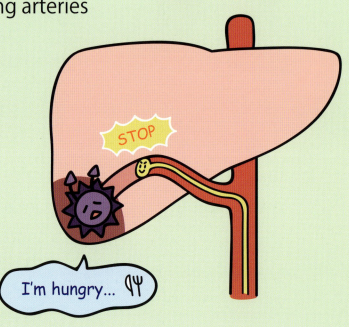

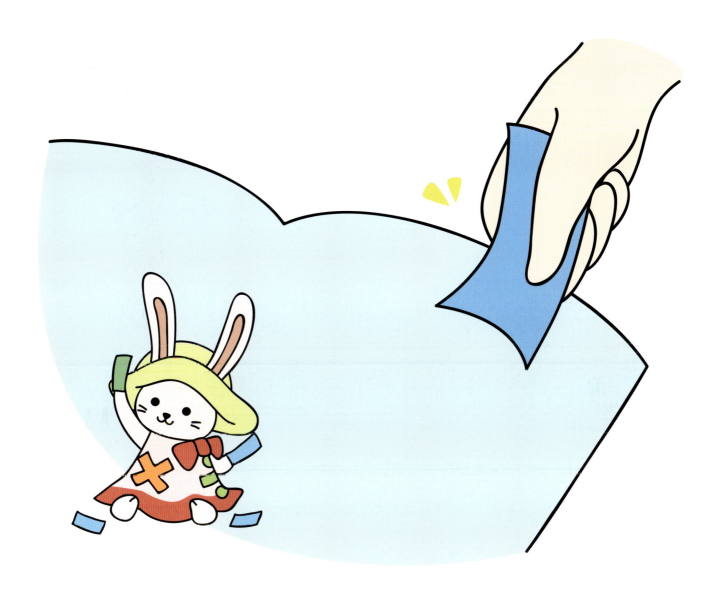

A person who saw a bookmark falling out of a book was the one who came up with the idea of a sticky note.

Weak glue ÷ Removable and reusable glue

⇒ **Sticky Note**

Question ①

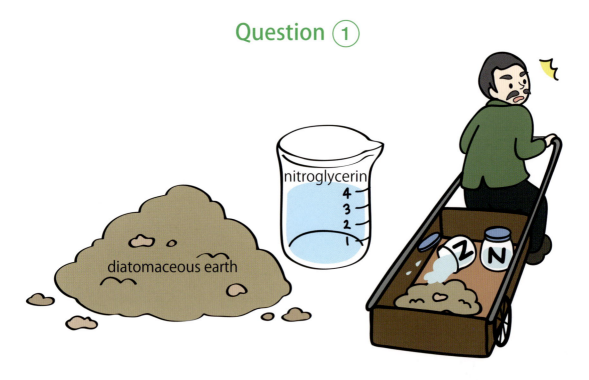

Invention of "Dynamite" Inventor：Alfred Nobel

Nobel developed a chemical substance called nitroglycerin. While carrying nitroglycerin in a container, the container cracked and the nitroglycerin leaked out. However, it was absorbed into diatomaceous earth (soil, used to prevent the containers from getting damaged) and did not explode. The soaking of nitroglycerin into diatomaceous earth and attaching a conductive wire led to the invention of dynamite that can be safely carried from one place to another.

※diatomaceous earth ＝ diatomite

Please fill in the following ☐ with the appropriate symbol ✚ ━ ✖ ➗ .

This invention came from the idea of

Question ②

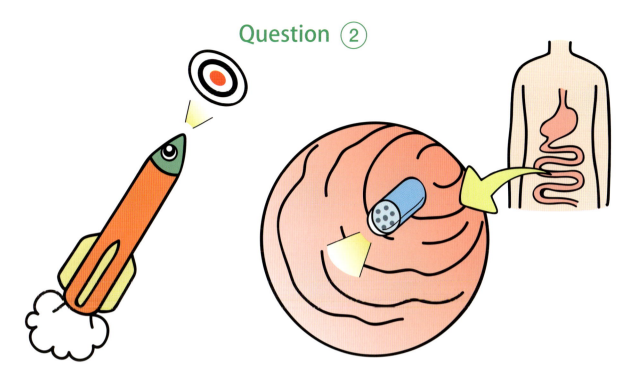

Invention of "Capsule Endoscope" Inventor : Gavriel Iddan

Iddan, who was working on developing a camera-equipped missile at the Ministry of Defense of Israel, met a gastroenterologist during his vacation in the United States in 1981 and came to know about the painful endoscopy examination. To make the examination easier, Iddan, came up with an idea of using miniaturized missiles in the endoscopy examination. In this way the capsule endoscope was invented in the form of "swallowable missiles".

Please fill in the following ☐ with the appropriate symbol ➕ ➖ ✖ ➗ .

This invention came from the idea of ☐ and ☐

Question ③

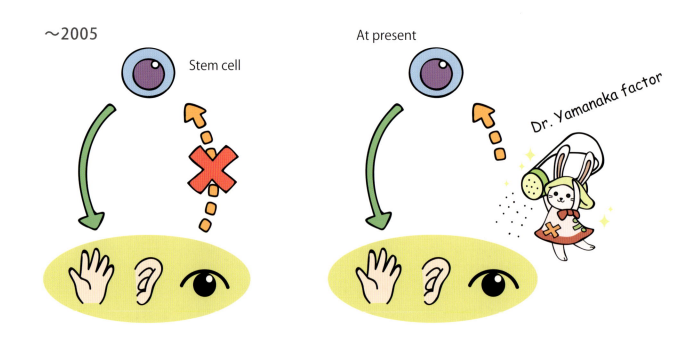

Invention of "iPS cell" Inventor：Shinya Yamanaka

Until 2005, it was believed that skin cells could never change into stem cells after differentiation. Introducing genes not only overturned this conventional wisdom, it also helped in the development of iPS cells, which can be transformed from skin cells into stem cells.

Please fill in the following □ with the appropriate symbol ✚ ━ ✖ ➗ .

This invention came from the idea of

Four Skills for Inventing

Inventions in General

Creative Implementatin
Addition

Development of **Pencil with Attached Eraser**

Eraser + Pencil

Development of **Dynamaite**

Nitroglycerin + Diatomaceous Earth

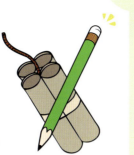

Efficient Streaming
Subtracting = Minimalizing

Development of **Fitness Footwear**

Slippers − Heels

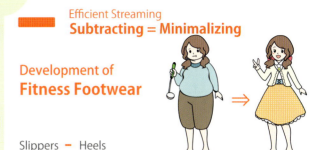

Lateral thinking
Multiplying = Recreating something in a different field

Development of **Refrigerator that keeps perishables longer**

Idea from a courier company ✕ Consumer electronics company

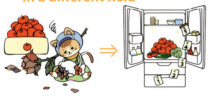

Overturns conventional wisdom
Dividing = Re-evaluating

Development of **the Sticky Note**

Weak glue ÷ Removable and reusable glue

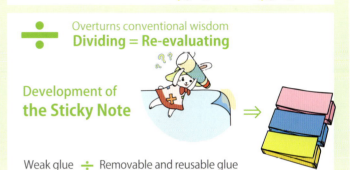

Inventions in the Medical Field

Creative Implementatin
Addition

Development of **the Magnifying Endoscope**

Endoscope
+
Microscope

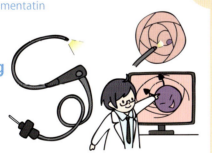

Efficient Streaming
Subtracting = Minimalizing

Development of the **Nasal Endoscope**

Endoscope
−
Having the thickness

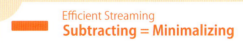
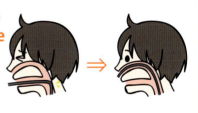

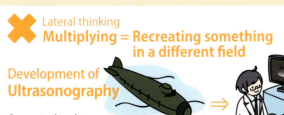

Lateral thinking
Multiplying = Recreating something in a different field

Development of **Ultrasonography**

Sonar technology used in military ships
✕
Medical field

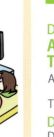

Overturns conventional wisdom
Dividing = Re-evaluating

Development of **Artery Embolization Treatment**

Arteries must not be clogged
÷
Treatment of cancer by clogging arteries

Development of **iPS Cells**
Differentiated cells ÷ Stem cells

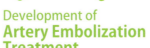
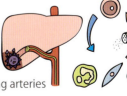

What is the difference between a discovery and an invention?

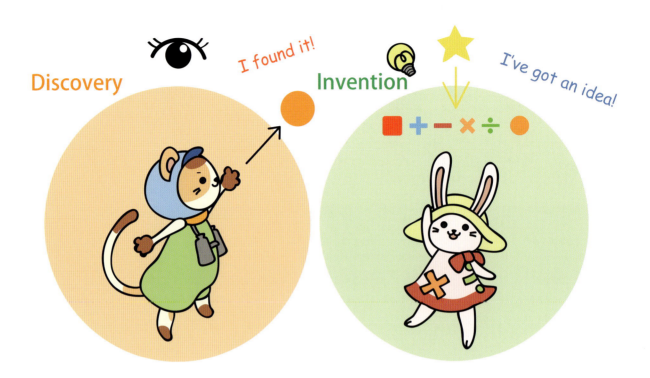

Everything you need for an invention is in yourselves!

A discovery is recognizing something that already exists for the first time, and that nobody has found before.

 Example：Isaac Newton discovered the Law of Gravitation.

An invention is creating something totally new with one's own ideas and experiences. Although an invention is completely new to the world, the physical materials needed for its production already exist, and just needs to be combined with the ideas and experiences of the individual. Utilizing all the materials with the skills of ✚ ━ ✖ and ➗ is what invention is all about. The combination of available materials has no limits.

 Example：Thomas Edison invented the phonograph, a machine to record and reproduce sound.

What kind of knowledge, skill and attitude do you want to develop from Hatsumeigaku?

Techniques
skills of ✚ ━ ✖ and ➗

Knowledge

All thoughts and ideas for an invention are in yourselves.

Readiness

In the field of observation, chance favors only the prepared mind.

(by Louis Pasteur)

By grasping and implementing there concepts, anyone could make an invention.

Correct answer

Question ①	✚	【Explanation】 Two different elements, nitroglycerin and diatomaceous earth, are combined together.
Question ②	✖ ━	【Explanation】 The use of an idea for military use in the medical field led to the miniaturization of huge missiles into swallowable capsules.
Question ③	➗	【Explanation】 iPS cells were developed from the idea of re-evaluating the idea that skin cells can be transformed into stem cells.

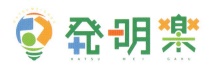

Epilogue

Each person has their own individual strengths. Some people might be good at sports, some others at cooking, and some might be good at painting. Even though, it sometimes seems like you have failed it can actually be a success. A person who changed the course of his/her life might feel somewhat lingering behind, however, nothing in life is wasted. All experiences are meaningful. In the world of invention, being different is worthy and gives joy.

(Acknowledgement)

This Book was published as a compilation of Hatsumeigaku classes at the Tottori University Hospital in 2012. The first edition was published in November 2012. Successively, the revised editions were published in April 2013 (2nd edition), March 2014 (3rd edition) and February 2016 (4th edition) as a part of a special funded project of the Ministry of Education, Culture, Sports, Science and Technology (MEXT) of Japan. Since the first publication, I have taught many classes at primary, junior high and high schools using this book as a textbook.

This time, we decided to make this book commercially available so that the concept of Hatsumeigaku can be learned by anyone who is interested. Inventing is a technique to combine your original materials and create something new whilst having fun. Everything you see or experienced can be used as materials for a new invention.

It is my hope that this book will serve as a textbook for those who are or may become interested in inventing things. Lastly, I would like to express my deepest appreciation to the MEXT of Japan, Kangaeru-gakkou and all those who in one way or another co-operated with this project.

Written by Masaru UEKI (Advanced Medicine, Innovation and Clinical Research Center, Tottori University Hospital)
Published in Japan by YAKUJI NIPPO, LTD., 1 Kanda Izumicho, Chiyoda-ku, Tokyo 101-8648.
www.yakuji.co.jp (online shop: yakuji-shop.jp)
Printed in Japan at FUJI REPRO, LTD.

© 2019 Tottori University Hospital. Any reproduction without permission is prohibited.

ISBN978-4-8408-1494-2